HEAL ME...PLEASE

Third Book in the LOVE ME, TOUCH ME, HEAL ME **Series**

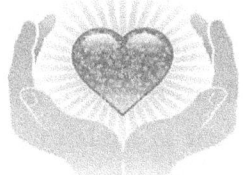

The Path to Physical, Emotional

Sexual and Spiritual Reawakening

Dr. Erica Goodstone

Copyright © 2009, Revised 2023   *Heal Me ... Please*   DrEricaGoodstone.com

Heal Me … Please is dedicated to

* Joel Goldsmith, whose Infinite Way teachings have cleared my spiritual blocks as I continually realize there is only one power
* Marian Strueken Bachmann, modern artist magnifique, who encouraged me many years ago to get my book published and invited me to her Infinite Way Group in NYC – and the rest is history.
* Tony Titshall, for opening his home so that a group of us can share and strengthen our connection to that one power together
* Sheila McKinney, for introducing me to Tony Titshall's group, and supporting me as I struggled to let go of my old beliefs and concepts
* Ken Lasdowski, for offering his loving insight, acceptance and joy of living that allowed me to accept my circumstances without resisting
* John Belnome, my friend and confidant, who allows me to share my concerns when the challenges of daily life threaten to disturb my peace of mind

Copyright © 2009, Revised 2023   *Heal Me … Please*   DrEricaGoodstone.com

Publisher Data & Legal Information

Copyright © 2009 Erica Goodstone, Ph.D. All rights reserved.
ISBN: 978-0-9824304-6-0
Published by Create Healing and Love Now Publishers
Contact the Publisher at : RelationshipHealingToolbox.com

All rights reserved. No part of this eBook may be reproduced, stored in a retrieval system or transmitted in any form or by any means electronic, mechanical, photocopying, recording, or oterhwise without express written permission of the author.

Every attempt has been made by the author to provide acknowledgement of the sources used for the material in this book. If there has been an omission of any source, please contact the author at
DrErica@DrEricaWellness.com

Disclaimer: No responsibility is assumed by the authors/publishers for any injury and/or damage and/or loss sustained in persons or property as a result of using this product; and/or for any liability, negligence or otherwise use or operation of any products, methods, instructions or ideas contained in the material herein.

The views and opinions expressed in this book and related materials are derived from the author's experience and research as a professor of health and physical education, yoga and meditation teacher, licensed mental health counselor, licensed professional counselor, licensed marriage and family therapist, board certified sex therapist, licensed massage and bodywork therapist, certified pain management practitioner, certified Integrative Medicine practitioner, certified Polarity Therapist, certified Rubenfeld Synergist, and involvement with numerous professional associations. She is not a licensed M.D. and does not diagnose or claim to cure any physical disease. She is also not a psychiatrist and does not claim to cure mental illness.

Any reader currently under the care or supervision of a psychiatrist, physician or other medical or behavioral health practitioner is urged to seek their professional advice before using or practicing any of the material or techniques contained herein.

Copyright © 2009, Revised 2023   *Heal Me … Please*   DrEricaGoodstone.com

ABOUT THE AUTHOR

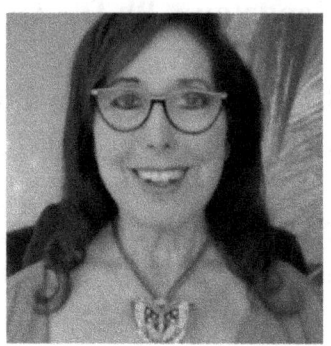

Erica Goodstone, Ph.D., has devoted her life's work to the discovery of love, healing and the creation of intimate, satisfying, fulfilling and joyful relationships. During over two decades, through her lectures, seminars and private counseling sessions, she has worked with thousands of men and women to create love and healing in their lives.

Having studied extensively from many different sources, Dr. Goodstone is a licensed mental health counselor, professional counselor, marriage and family therapist, massage and bodywork therapist. She is a diplomate and fellow for the American Association of Integrative Medicine and a diplomate for the American Academy of Pain Management. Dr. Goodstone is also a diplomate for the American Board of Sexology, a fellow for the American Academy of Clinical Sexologists, and a certified Sex Therapist for the American Association of Sexuality Educators and Therapists.

As a former professor of health and physical education at F.I.T./State University of New York, Dr. Goodstone spent 25 years studying and teaching about the body: physical fitness, health and wellness, stress management, sports psychology, team building and human sexuality. But she did not stop there.

Dr. Goodstone also spent many years studying a wide variety of healing body therapy modalities in including massage, shiatsu, polarity therapy, craniosacral therapy, Reiki, reflexology, Chinese medical theory, Japanese healing theories. Her studies led to the combination of touch with counseling through the gentle yet profound Rubenfeld Synergy

Method. In fact, she was on the original steering committee and the board of directors for the first two terms of the U.S. Association for Body Psychotherapy. This was the first organization to bring together all the different originators and practitioners of somatic body psychotherapy methods and modalities.

But Dr. Goodstone's knowledge and background does not stop there. She has also fervently and passionately craved her own inner spiritual development and outer social awareness. Her seeking led her to spend many years studying yoga, first with the Sivananda Center in New York City and at the Sivananda Ashram in Paradise Island, Bahamas, where she met Swami Vishnu Devananda and listened to Ravi Shankar play the sitar. Later she spent years working with Guru Mayi, Swami Muktananda's disciple, receiving Darshan and personal counseling as needed.

Her studies included attending many consciousness raising seminars in the 1980's, including the EST seminars led by Werner Erhard, the Living Love Workshops led by Ken Keyes, Jr., author of *The Handbook to Higher Consciousness,* and DMA seminars about the creative process and structural thinking led by Robert Fritz.
She avidly studied the Rosicrucian manuals for many years, along with the Kaballah teachings of The Builders of the Adytum and the Course in Miracles. Her current focus has been exclusively upon the works of Joel Goldsmith, *The Infinite Way*, and Siddha Yoga Master Swami Muktananda..

Dr. Erica Goodstone has been a celebrated speaker at national and local professional and public events. Since her doctoral dissertation, which studied the effects of early mother-infant bonding upon later adult intimacy, she has continued to write extensively about creating love through the healing power of touch, intimacy, and the mind/body/spirit connection.

Dr. Goodstone's interviews and articles have appeared in *Who's Who of Medicine and Healthcare, CBS 4 TV, Blog Talk Radio Logical Soul Talk, Mademoiselle, Cosmopolitan , Marie Claire, Penthouse Forum, Journal of Sex and Marital therapy, Newsletters of the U.S. Association for Body Psychotherapy.* Dr. Goodstone has a very wide presence on the web. Her bio and blogs appear on numerous sites, e.g., Wordpress.com and Gather.com, as well as numerous ezines, most notably ezinearticles.com,

Dr. Goodstone's chapter, "Sexual Reawakening appears in the wonderfully organized book of Rubenfeld Synergy practitioners, *Healing Journeys: The Power of Rubenfeld Synergy, V. Mechner, Ed.* She has also written a section about touch therapies in the internationally acclaimed book, *The Continuum Complete International Encyclopedia of Sexuality*, R. J Noonan and R. Francoeur, Eds.

Dr. Goodstone can be reached at DrErica@DrEricaWellness.com

****

INTRODUCTION To The Series

Love Me, Touch Me, Heal Me: The Path to Physical, Emotional, Sexual and Spiritual Reawakening shows us what it takes to love, touch, and heal our own self. As we heal, we develop a renewed passion for life, a deep sense of being connected to something beyond our immediate life circumstances, and an increased desire for intimate loving. *Love Me, Touch Me, Heal Me* is meant to be a coming out party, coming out of hiding, bringing our total self into the light for examination, acceptance, and readiness to share our authentic self intimately with others.

Clients, colleagues and friends have often asked me to recommend a good book about love and relationships or about emotional intimacy and sexual communication. Others have requested information about ways to heal their body through natural methods, e.g., diet, exercise, body therapy, or even spirituality. And some have wondered what the best psychological approach might be to overcome fears, anxiety, anger, depression or relationship conflicts.

Answers to the above questions will be easily obtained as you read through this series of four ebooks. You will discover that you can find the answers to most of your problems, dilemmas, life issues and concerns through self-evaluation. As you complete the exercises, you will literally begin to heal your cellular memories, create new brain patterns and remove lifelong blocks to intimate joyful relating. You can turn to professionals for expert opinions, guidance, support and mentoring, but with this book you will begin to more fully trust your own inner knowing about what is truly best for your growth and healing.

FORMAT OF THIS BOOK

This **Book Series** is divided into four books consisting of three chapters in each book as follows:

Book I   **Love Me … Please**

    Chapter 1   The Gift of Love
    Chapter 2   Be Who You Are…The Greatest Gift of All
    Chapter 3   The Delicate Dance of Love

Book II   **Touch Me … Please**

    Chapter 1   Your Body Believes You
    Chapter 2   It's a Sensational World
    Chapter 3   Touching Matters…The Profound Effects of Body Therapy

Book III   **Heal Me … Please**

    Chapter 1   Heal Me…Please
    Chapter 2   Let All Your Senses Speak…As You Heal
    Chapter 3   Touching Stories…Healing Through Body Psychotherapy

Book IV   **Sexual and Spiritual Reawakening**

    Chapter 1   Ordinary People, Ordinary/Extraordinary Sex
    Chapter 2   Ten Simple Steps to Sexual Reawakening
    Chapter 3   Sexual And Spiritual Reawakening…At Last

- Every chapter contains vital information, theories, concepts and suggestions gleaned from years of study, research, personal and professional experiences.

- Every chapter includes pertinent real-life stories, individual and partner written, verbal and contemplative exercises.

- Every chapter builds upon the previous one in the healing process.

- Every chapter is also complete unto itself.

- You may choose to read one entire book from start to finish and then begin a second book.

- You may choose to start with a specific chapter in any of the books.

- Resources, references, and keywords will appear at the end of each book.

This entire series of four books was originally intended to be one book. Written many years ago, this book has been hibernating in file boxes until now, a time when this world needs all the love we can muster. And this book teaches us how.

Love Me, Touch Me, Heal Me: The Path to Physical, Emotional, Sexual and Spiritual Reawakening belongs in the personal library of anyone who truly wants to heal from the past and create loving, touching and authentically intimate relationships. This is a guidebook, a reference book, and a comforting friend along the path to reawakening.

HOW TO USE THIS BOOK

This book is about your life, my life, and all of our lives. Read this book, follow the exercises, and watch miracles happen. *Love Me, Touch Me, Heal Me* is a life transforming healing process. For best results, you will need a few basic materials.

1. **<u>Writing Materials</u>**

    a. **A journal, preferably a beautiful, special journal, but any 4" by 6" or 8" by 10" lined or unlined, notebook will do.** Choosing a journal or notebook that is special to you creates an experience of sensory stimulation every time you write in it! If you choose to write all the exercises in this book on pieces of paper, that's okay. But, if the outer appearance is appealing and soothing to your eyes, if the texture satisfies your sense of touch, if there's a fragrance of fresh cut paper or soft smooth leather that comforts you, the power of the words you write will be enhanced. Your brain will connect the sensual beauty of your journal with your written words and with your life. Your mind and body will begin to believe that you are serious about creating healing, love, spiritual connection, sexual aliveness, and joy in your life.

b. **Pen, pencil, colored pencils or crayons.**

Brain research indicates that the mind absorbs information best when all the senses are involved. So get yourself a box of colored pencils, colored pens or crayons. You'll probably discover that you want some pastels, and maybe even paint and brushes before you're through. Colors and textures add additional dimensionality to your writing, increasing the possibility for your brain to record and store your hopes and dreams, uplifting words, goals, new beliefs, and appropriate affirmations. This allows your mind, at a later point in time, to easily refute your fears, frustrations and anxieties as they arise in your consciousness. Crayons and colored pencils may also stimulate your brain to create images, faces, doodles, and other self-expressions that reveal some important subconscious personal thought

Processes.

2. *A quiet place, even a corner of a room, set aside to practice the exercises.*

Energy accumulates in a space that you set aside and use specifically for one purpose. Creating a special place for your own inner work is a strong suggestion to your subconscious, (the part of your brain that allows your dreams to germinate into fruition), that you are serious about transforming your life.

3. *Recording Materials*

Choose your own recording device.

To do the exercises in this book, you can read and stop, read and stop, or you can record your own voice first. Then you will be able to go straight through the exercise without stopping. The goal is for you to comfort yourself and love yourself. Hearing your own voice is a powerful affirmation that you can create what you want and you are all you will ever truly need.

As you begin your journey along the path to love, take a moment to assess where you are right now in your life. The questions you are about to answer may seem simple but are actually quite profound. Observe your thoughts. Notice any automatic body responses you may have. You are more than your thoughts. You are more than your body. Allow your automatic responses to help you to discover who you truly are.

For all the exercises in this introduction and in the rest of this book, you have choices. You can read the exercise and then write in your journal. You can record the entire exercise with your own voice, close the book, close your eyes, and visualize freely. Or, you can listen to the pre-recorded audio tapes that accompany each chapter.

Who Are You?

Sit in a comfortable position.

Inhale slowly, very slowly, and deeply.

Exhale slower than your usual rate.

Take three slow, deep, easy, and quiet breaths.

Close your eyes and allow your body to relax.

Take three more slow, deep, easy, and quiet breaths.

Open your eyes only to read each question.

Immediately close your eyes and allow the answer to come to you.

Accept the answers that come. Do not edit or change the response

Listen to your mind's first answer, the most correct response at this moment.

> *Who am I?*
>
> *What are other people here for in my life?*
>
> *Why am I alive now?*
>
> *What do I believe about love?*
>
> *Who do I enjoy touching and for what purpose?*
>
> *What yearns to heal inside of me?*
>
> *What does sexual reawakening mean to me?*
>
> *What is the role of God, a higher power, or spirituality in my life?*

Copyright © 2009, Revised 2023   *Heal Me … Please*   DrEricaGoodstone.com

TABLE OF CONTENTS

PART THREE   *HEAL ME ... PLEASE*

Introduction To The Series....................7
   Format of The Book
   How To Use This Book
   Who Are You?

Table of Contents............................16

***Heal Me ... Please* Introduction**..............21
   Healing Happens In Every Moment...................22
   Heal Me Please Poem...........................25

Chapter 1   *HEAL ME ... PLEASE*..............27

   Oh My Aching Back..............................27
      The People You Have Loved
      The People Who Have Loved You
      How Have You Loved Yourself?
      Your Suffering
      Forgiving Yourself And Others
      Where Is Your Passion?
   The Healing Power of Love........................37
      Your House Pets
      Love Your Body As Your Most Precious Pet
      How Have You Been Treating Your Body?
      A Family Affair
      How Have You Been Treating Your Body?
   When Your Body Is Healthy.......................43
      The Hospital Bed
      Life Is Precious
      Lessons From Your Illness

Copyright © 2009, Revised 2023   *Heal Me ... Please*   DrEricaGoodstone.com

How Have Your Health Practitioners Treated You?
Your Healing History
Your Healing Needs
Your Health Habits Inventory

Change and Healing..51
Your Health Investment Portfolio
Return On Your Health Investments
Your Commitment To Healing

What Does God Mean To You?..............................56
Following Your Own Spiritual Path
What Does God Have To Do With Your Healing?
Your Connection To God
The Joy Of Suffering

Chapter 2 LET ALL YOUR SENSES SPEAK AS YOU HEAL......................63

Touch Me Today Poem........................63

Let Your Senses Speak To You.........................65
What Are Your Five Senses Revealing?
Reawakening Through Sensual Awareness

What Do You See?..69
Open Your Eyes and See
Judge What Your Eyes See
Set Your Sights

Do You Hear What I Hear?...................................74
Open Your Ears and Listen
How Do You Listen To Yourself?
How Do You Listen To Others?
What Do You Hear When You Listen?
What Are Your Listening And Speaking Goals?

Open Your Sense Of Smell..........................79
Breathing
Smelling

Open Your Sense Of Taste............................83
Taste Your World

Open Your Sense Of Touch..........................84
Touch Your World

Chapter 3   TOUCHING STORIES
HEALING THROUGH TOUCH AND BODY PSYCHOTHERAPY......89
The Story Of My Life Poem……………….....89

Touching Stories……………………………………...91
- George's Handshake
- Lana's Unconsummated Marriage
- The Revitalization of Steve's Life
- The Truth About John
- Carol's Vagina Speaks
- Louis's Panic Attacks
- Henry's Tears

What Is Body Psychotherapy?..............................108
- How Does The Body Psychotherapy Process Work?
- Body Psychotherapy Allows Us To Breathe In Life
- Body Psychotherapy Energizes Our Brain
- Body Psychotherapy Reveals And Uncovers Our Truth
- Body Psychotherapy Helps Us To Heal
- Body Psychotherapy Reopens Our Heart To Love
- Body Psychotherapy Reawakens Our Sensual, Sexual and Spiritual Aliveness
- Body Psychotherapy Reconnects Us To Our Soul
- Body Psychotherapy Reminds Us To Play

A Body Psychotherapy Session…………………..117
- Your Body's Messages
- Body Psychotherapy Clears The Path For Love, Relationships and Intimacy

More To Come…………………………………123

Also by Dr. Erica Goodstone…………………….127

HEAL ME ... PLEASE

BOOK THREE

Heal Me ... Please, Book Three, is dedicated to

- Joel Goldsmith, whose *Infinite Way* teachings have cleared my spiritual blocks as I continually realized there is only one power
- Marian Streuken Bachmann, modern artist Magnifique, who encouraged me many years ago to get my book published and invited me to my first *Infinite Way* group at her home in NYC – and the rest is history
- Tony Titshall, for opening his home so that a dedicated group of us can share and strengthen our connection to that one power together
- Sheila McKinney, for introducing me to Tony Titshall's group, and supporting me as I struggled to let go og my old beliefs and concepts
- Ken Lasdowski, for offering his loving insight, acceptance and joy of living that allowed me to more easily accept my current circumstances without resisting
- John Delnome, my friend and confidant, who allows me to share my concerns when the challenges of daily life threaten to disturb my peace of mind.

INTRODUCTION

Heal me … please

Why me? Why this? Why now?

Heal me, please

What will you do to me?

Heal me, please

What will I have to do?

Heal me … please.

Erica Goodstone, Ph.D. 1/29/00

Healing Happens In Every Moment

Healing happens in every moment, in every cell and organ of our body. Loving, touching, and being touched with love, we heal. When we heal, our bodies relax and our lives come into balance. In healing, we discover our own truth, face our inner spirit, and we begin to know God.

In **Heal Me ... Please**, the third book in this four part series, we examine the healing process: what we believe about healing, how we have healed our self and others, and how we can create healing in our bodies, our intimate relationships, our sexuality, and our lives. You will discover what it takes to heal whatever ails you. You will look at what has helped you to heal and what has hindered your healing in the past. Through writing exercises and closed eye meditations, you will discover new ways to connect with and stimulate your own healing presence within.

Together we will examine our sensual responses, the healing messages revealed to us through our senses, and ways to enhance our sensual responsiveness. As you increase your own sensual awareness, you will naturally become more readily attuned to the unique sensual responsiveness of everyone, including your most intimate partners.

Through stories of real people's lives, we explore the life transforming, healing potential of touch and body psychotherapy. These stories are excerpts of actual case histories, therapy sessions, emotional responses, and eventual healing that took place in seminars and private sessions. Of course, names and identifying personal characteristics have been altered to protect anonymity. None of my clients will be able to say with certainty, "That's me!" Yet, as you read these stories, you may recognize something familiar within yourself. You may even identify with some of these clients' experiences.

We are all voyagers on a life path back to wholeness. Many of us tend to focus on our problems and the possible causes, recalling in detail the many ways we may have felt wronged. In this book we turn our focus toward healing our problems, letting them go, and moving toward creating what we truly desire.

****

HEAL ME ... PLEASE

"Heal Thyself and Do No Harm"

Hippocratic Dictum

Healing happens in every moment, in every cell and organ of our body. When we love and are touched with love, we heal. When we heal, our body relaxes and our life come into balance. When we heal, we discover our own truth, we face our inner spirit, and we begin to know God. In Part III, we examine the healing process: what we believe about healing, how we have healed our self and others, and how we can create healing in our body, our intimate relationships, our sexuality, and our life.

HEAL ME ... PLEASE

Heal Me ... Please

I came to you
Lost in despair
You took me in
With open arms
Welcome
My darling friend
Soul mate
On the path
To unconditional love
Acceptance
Being
Human Be-ing
My words came pouring out
Flooding the room
Intensifying
Exploding
Subsiding
Softening
Subdued

My spirit calmed down
I felt safe
Connected
Affected
Protected
Loved
You listened
Open arms
You spoke
Open heart

My troubled spirit
Found its home
Inside myself
Again

Copyright © 8/27/97 Erica Goodstone, Ph.D.

HEAL ME … PLEASE

CHAPTER 1

HEAL ME … PLEASE

Oh My Aching Back!

Lying on the floor. Cold. Frightened. Unable to move. The last time I looked at the clock it was 10:30 A.M. The time now was 2 P.M. Moving or turning even slightly was excruciating, sending my body into a contraction, shooting pain up and down my spine. It all happened because of overexerting my self, pushing beyond my limits, not paying attention to the messages my body was loudly sending (spasms, pain – take it easy) then accidentally falling off a chair. I prayed to God, "Please help me get up." Another hour passed.

Wondering, "What can I do to help myself, I suddenly thought of reflexology. The only body parts I could move without causing unbearable pain were my fingers. Desperate, I pressed the fingers of my right hand along the outer edge of the palm of my left hand in the area corresponding to the spine of my back.. Then I used my left hand to press the same area on the palm of my right hand and fingers. Miraculously, in a little while, I was able to maneuver my body ever so slowly to position my back so that it was facing a portable heater that happened to be on the floor nearby. Finally, I was close enough to turn the heater on. Eventually, the heat relaxed my contracted back muscles just enough for me to manage to stand up. Standing felt like paradise to me.

While lying on the floor for 4 1/2 hours, I prayed to God and my angels to please help me get up and get to a doctor. I believe they were there assisting me, but they had to be sure I would use all of my own resources first. I had the terrifying thought, "What if the pain never ends? What if I can never walk and move and exercise and enjoy life's activities again?"

Every one of us is vulnerable to the unpredictability and randomness of life. Now is the time to face and get on with our life; now, at this moment, while we still have most of our senses and most of our physical, emotional and mental abilities intact. Without warning, we can suddenly meet with extreme good fortune or unanticipated disaster. The untimely deaths (through plane crashes, automobile accidents, murders, assassinations, and other tragedies) people we hear about in the news, or perhaps our own personal experiences, have reminded us again and again about the fragility and preciousness of life.

Many of us complain bitterly and continuously about our life, not realizing that when we have our health and most of our senses are working adequately, we truly have everything we need. If we have lost our lover, failed in school, been fired from a job, or abused by our spouse or parents, as long as we have our senses and our mind, we can re-create our life to fulfill our dreams. As long as we are alive, it is never too late to heal.

Healing happens in every moment of our life. Cells die. Cells regenerate. New cells are born. In fact, we actually have a totally new body, all of our cells replaced with new cells, every seven years. Our immune system continuously works to ward off foreign invaders. But the ultimate healing happens when we are ready to face our Creator, when our body prepares us for physical death. As we die, our body unwinds, letting go of all the stress that binds us, releasing the emotional and physical habit patterns that have ruled our life.

I remember my polarity therapy colleague, Ray, poignantly describing a polarity session with his aging mother. He cradled her head in his open hands, his index fingers gently resting against the sides of her neck in a position that creates a sense of well-being, safety, feeling nurtured and loved. As he held her head, his mother breathed her final breath.

Ray continued to hold her head, pausing only briefly to dial 911. As the emergency crew arrived, Ray observed that, even after his mother was no longer breathing and her heart had stopped beating, her energy continued to unwind. In his gentle grasp, he felt his mother's head and neck, which had always been stiff and almost immovable, beginning to give way in his hands, to soften and to move easily from side to side. As he held his mother's head, he watched her emotional burdens vanish before his eyes. The stress lines on her face diminished and almost disappeared. Her face took on an innocent, child-like, almost angelic appearance. Ray felt assured that her chronic human problems had been removed, that she was healed and at peace and ready to face her creator.

Many people who have been pronounced dead, whose hearts actually stopped beating, claim to have had life transforming experiences. Many have seen a dark tunnel and a bright light, some say they have met with spiritual beings, deceased family members, and old friends. Not everyone who nearly died saw the same visions or felt the same feelings. However, most of these people came to realize that nothing in this lifetime is more important than love. Nothing surpasses love.

- **Believing is receiving.**
- **Believe in love.**
- **Believe in the power of love to heal.**
- **Watch miracles happen.**

The People You Have Loved

Sit quietly and close your eyes. Take a few slow, deep, easy breaths. Now, think about the people you have loved. For each person you have loved, ask the following questions:

What about this person touched my heart and caused me to feel love?

Would I love this person if I first met him or her now? Why?

What did I believe this person could offer me or do for you?

Was I satisfied or disappointed?

How did I respond?

What did I believe I could offer that person?

The People Who Have Loved You

Recall the people who have loved you.

For each person who has loved you, ask the following questions:

What about me touched their heart and caused them to feel love?

Would this person love me if he or she met me now? Why?

What did they believe I could offer them or do for them?

Were they satisfied or disappointed?

How did they respond?

What did I believe they could offer me?

How Have You Loved Your Self?

At the top of one page write: *How I Have Loved Myself.* Make a list of the ways you have shown concern and love for yourself, attempted to satisfy your own needs and desires, put your own needs before the needs and requests of others in the distant past, the recent past and in your current life. At the top of a second page write: *How I Have Not Loved Myself.* List the ways you have disregarded yourself, ignored your own needs and desires, put others' needs and requests before your own in the distant past, the recent past and in your current life.

How many of us are right here, right now, existing in a place of our own choosing where we can suffer? Some of us have been taught that life is hard, that we don't deserve to feel good, that feeling good is actually bad, or that if we allow our self to feel good, something bad will surely follow. If we believe life is hard, even at those times when it is easy, we will probably find a way to make life difficult. On the other hand, some of us believe that life and people *should* be easy or *should* be a certain way. If we believe life should be easy, when we fall into difficult circumstances, we will probably suffer more than the situation calls for.

Your Suffering

Who or what in your life do you believe has caused you to suffer?
Make a list of every person or situation, including God and including yourself, who you believe has caused you to suffer. Begin with, *"It's his/her fault that ...."* Here's you chance to point a finger and to blatantly blame

everything and everyone in your life who you believe has caused you to suffer. When you finish your blame list, answer the following questions:

Where and how did you learn about the way life is and the way people are?

Did you learn that you are good, worthy and deserving?

Did you learn that others are good, worthy and deserving?

In what ways have you interfered with attaining, having, and keeping what you want?

In what ways have you created and participated in your own suffering?

Most of us have not learned to face life as it is. We develop faulty ideas about the way we think our lives *should* be. Often, we have unrealistic and unfair expectations about the way other people *should* be, *should* feel, *should* behave. Sometimes we are unrealistically optimistic about the potential of others, choosing to see them the way we would like them to be instead of truly seeing who they are. Sometimes we make comparisons between the way we live and the way others appear to be living. When our lives seem to be less than the way we perceive others' lives to be, we may become anxious and demanding and actually, through our own actions, sabotage the good that we do have.

Forgiving Yourself and Others

At the top of one page write, *People I Have Not Forgiven.* List the names of those you have not been able to forgive.

What interferes with my ability or desire to forgive this person or persons?

What would have to happen for me to be able to forgive this person or persons?

At the top of a second page write, *What I Have Not Forgiven Myself For?* List the traits or actions you have been unable to forgive yourself for having or doing.

What interferes with my ability or desire to forgive myself?

What would have to happen for me to be able to forgive myself?

Forgiveness is one of the most powerful tools we have in our possession at all times. Just as we can suddenly experience extreme good fortune or extreme disaster, we can just as suddenly choose to forgive a person, place or situation. Forgiving ourselves and others helps us to heal. If we harbor feelings of being an unfortunate victim, of having been irrevocably harmed, of believing that someone or something is unworthy of God's love, we eventually hurt ourselves. Forgiveness is not to please or heal others. Forgiveness heals our own lives. No matter what has happened in the past, when we choose to forgive, our minds and our hearts become more receptive to love. We revive our joy in living and once again discover our true passion.

Where Is Your Passion?

What activities or goals create excitement and passion for you?

What activities or goals keep your mind focused?

What activities, for you, would be dream adventures?

What activities would you like to share with others?

What activities would you prefer to do alone?

What personal traits, emotions, people or situations in your life have interfered with feeling your passion and pursuing those activities that you feel passionate about?

What would it take to rekindle your passion for life?

The Healing Power of Love

There is nothing more real and more powerful than love. We can feel The reverberation of love in every cell of our body. Physicists have measured heart energy. Heart transplant recipients learn the language of the heart, their own and that of their heart donor.

Dis-ease, physical or psychological, is often a sign that we have been ignoring, abusing, neglecting, avoiding or actually hating a part of us. Many of us neglect to take care of our body's needs for nourishing food, regular and proper exercise, good body mechanics, postural alignment, sleep, and relaxation. Our body may tolerate this situation for awhile. In time, however, our body parts will break down.

We may have been indulging in sexual activity without intimacy or commitment, ignoring and denying our heart's need for loving connection. Over time, our heart's message will reach the brain which may signal to our pituitary, the master gland, to stop producing hormones that stimulate desire and lead to orgasm. Our sexual organs, in response to our heart's message, may finally decide to give up the fight and shut down.

All of our organs share the same network of blood and blood vessels, lymph and lymph vessels, nerves, muscles, glands, connective tissue, fat and skin. They all need to receive fresh oxygen from the lungs. Spend a moment to contemplate the holographic nature of our amazing mind-body-spiritual system. Can you fathom that this whole system functions as one cohesive unit of love?

Without love and touch and stimulation, infants as well as the elderly become depressed, chronically ill, and eventually die. Even animals die without love and attention. A friend of mine had two wonderful cats. One summer, while she traveled, she left her two cats home alone, one and off, for a period of two months. She left plenty of food and water for them and she returned once every week or two to check in on them and repack her bags. On one of her visits to her home, she found the older cat lying dead in the middle of her living room. After burying the cat, she went off on another trip. When she returned home a week later, she found her other cat had also died. My friend learned a painful lesson she will never forget. Both of her cats died from lack of love and touch and nurturing.

Your House Pets

Do you have a pet?

If not, why have you chosen not to have a pet?

What type of pet/s would you get if your circumstances allowed for it, cat, dog, bird, fish, horse, monkey, other?

How do you believe this pet could benefit your life and your health?

If you do have a pet or several pets, explain why you have chosen to have a pet and why you have selected the particular pet/s.

What type of pet/s do you have?

What factors influenced your choice?

How do your pets show their love?

How do you show love toward your pet/s?

What type of pet/s would you get if your circumstances allowed for it, cat, dog, bird, fish, other?

How do you believe this pet could benefit your life and your health?

Why would you choose to have a cat or a dog as your pet? They require care, attention, time, and money. They restrict your freedom and curtail your travel and other activities. Research shows that people with pets are happier, healthier and less stressed. Why? Cats and dogs emanate pure love. They live in the moment and they love unconditionally. They respond to your nonverbal cues. They respond to your mood swings and emotions. They feel deeply and love you completely.

Love Your Body As Your Most Precious Pet

Love your body. Honor it. Nurture it. Be gentle with it. Train it to perform at optimum levels for you. Give it rest. Allow it to relax. Give it rewards - lots of rewards, frequently, at regular intervals. Talk kindly to your body. Listen to its messages. Pay attention to your body just the way a caring mother listens to the sounds of her newborn infant.

Your body's messages are loud and clear, not subtle. Many of us have blocked our hearing, refusing to listen. Ignoring our body's messages and signals will not make the problems go away. They may go into hiding. The signals may get softer and more difficult to decipher. The problems may go deeper and become more pervasive, spreading to distant parts of your body.

Candace Pert's ground breaking scientific research on neuropeptides reveals that our bodies do, indeed, function as an integrated network system. Her studies show that information is stored, processed and exchanged through information carriers known as neuropeptides. These special substances are stored in the bone marrow, the place where immune cells develop. Neuropeptides have receptor sites in many different parts of the brain and in our body organs. Hormones and neuropeptides are also distributed throughout the body through the master gland, the pituitary, located at the base of the brain.

The ignored body parts or organs may lay dormant, isolated and neglected for a long time, perhaps years and even decades. However, at some point, your organs will begin to seek attention, each organ fighting for control. Imagine that? Imagine your mind demanding respect, your heart crying for compassion, your liver raging to eliminate its negative debris, your lungs gasping for more breathing room, and your stomach filling your abdominal cavity against the will of your intestines.

In a happy, cohesive family everyone has a chance to thrive. But, if family members are upset, fighting with each other, and become distant and isolated, each person is affected. Isn't it much wiser for family members to talk to each other privately, regularly, and sometimes at family meetings to air any grievances, and to reinforce the love of happy family life. Our bodies, when healthy, function like one big happy family. But when communication between our body cells breaks down, we become like a dysfunctional family, our individual organs starving for love and nourishment.

A FAMILY AFFAIR

Bring your body to your own family party. Let all your internal members greet each other, hug and have a quiet conversation. Let each part express its needs, desires, dreams and feelings. Let each part respond to every other part. Imagine all your organs and body parts having a meeting where they make an agreement to listen and respect one another's needs. In your journal, list the statements your body parts agree are essential for the healthy functioning of your entire bodily organization.

How Have You Been Treating Your Body?

How have you been treating your body as the container and home of your internal family?

How have you been treating each of your body organs?

Have you maintained contact with every part of your body?

Have you ignored or responded to your body's messages?

Have you handled problems by cutting out the offending body part, removing it, sending it away?

What has been the effect of actions you have taken toward your own body?

When Your Body Is Healthy

When your body is healthy, your emotions stable, and your five senses working, you expect you will always remain this way. Most of us don't realize that in one instant, any moment, our lives can change dramatically. A car accident, a sports injury, even an accidental fall can leave us bedridden, or walking around with unsightly bandages or a clumsy back or neck brace. Suddenly we may become self-conscious and inhibited, feeling disabled and different. In our Marlboro Man, Super Woman, Body Piercing society, being physically challenged, ill, or dependent on others, is not okay.

There but for the grace of God go I. Every one of us is vulnerable to the unpredictability and randomness of life. Without warning, on any day of our lives, we can meet with mild or extreme good fortune or life-threatening disaster.

The Hospital Bed

Close your eyes. Imagine you have just awakened from a deep sleep. Nurses are standing nearby. The doctor who examined you asks, in a concerned voice, *"How are you feeling?"* All you feel is groggy, sleepy and bewildered. You don't know why you're here or where you are. The doctor explains, "You were in a terrible accident. We didn't think you were going to make it. You must have a strong will to live." You want to sit up. That's when you realize, *"I can't move. I want to talk but the words won't come out. A tear drips down your face."* The doctor notices and tells you the words you are dreading. *"You are paralyzed from head to toe. You have a rare condition called "Locked in Syndrome."* We see that your right eye tears and your eyelid opens and closes. We will set up a special gadget for you. By moving your right eye, and selecting letters of the alphabet, you will be able to communicate with us.

Sound farfetched and not possible? Two astounding books were written by victims of this horrible affliction. Using only the blinking of his left eye, Jean-Dominique Bauby, editor in chief of *French Elle*, selected letters of the alphabet to write a book about his ordeal. Julia Tayson Tavalaro, a beautiful, happily married, 32 year old woman, living in her dream home with her beloved husband and 14 month old daughter, after a series of sudden strokes, was only able to make small movements with her head, neck and eyes and eventually some groaning, grunting sounds. A specially constructed pointer attached to her head allowed her to select letters, one by one, to write lengthy poems and complete her memoirs.

Life Is Precious

Life is precious. Every moment counts. Savor every moment. Ken Keyes, author of *The Handbook for Higher Consciousness* (Living Love Center, 1975), tells a beautiful story about living in the moment. *A young man in the jungle, pursued by a tiger, quickly climbs a tree. The tiger rapidly approaching, the young man is hanging onto a branch that he knows is about to break off the tree. At that moment, he notices a beautiful, ripe strawberry. As his branch is breaking and he is about to meet his fate in the jaws of the hungry tiger below, the young man reaches out, plucks the strawberry, eats it, and enjoys the sweet taste.*

That young man was living in the moment, enjoying the most that was possible even as he faced a certain death. Perhaps you have personally experienced a devastating physical illness. Perhaps you are currently living with chronic physical or emotional problems, that may never go away. If you are currently in a physically challenged state, how are you handling it? What are you telling yourself and others? A useful thought for you might be: **It is not what life hands us that counts, but what we do with the life we are handed.** A beautiful healing statement that someone wrote is: *Life is not freedom from the storm but peace within the storm.*

For those of us currently living in good health, imagine how you might cope if your active, healthy life came to a screaming halt, unexpectedly? Would you wallow in self-pity, anger, rage and helplessness? Would you slide through the center of a crowded subway clanking a jar of coins, begging total strangers to give you money for having no legs? I saw such a man, groveling in the midst of stressed out, disinterested working people.

As long as we are healthy, we can choose to ignore body signals, the meaning of life, and the purpose of relationships. We can ignore the power of love. However, no matter how much pride and self-sufficiency our ego pretends to have, when we become ill we need other people -- doctors, nurses, close family members, friends, neighbors, or acquaintances.

Becoming ill interferes with our normal routine in life. We are forced to curtail our activities, sometimes to remain perfectly still in bed for an indefinite period of time. During that quiet time, we have an opportunity to review our lives and to learn lessons that our illness can teach us.

Lessons From Your Illness

Remember a time when you were ill. That time could be right now. If you are currently ill, use your current situation for this exercise. Write a brief memoir of your illness.

Describe your illness.

Where were you when you first became ill?

Who was there with you at first and as the illness progressed?

How did that person treat you and how did you feel about that?

What were your told about your illness? By whom?

Did you ignore or deny your illness for any length of time? What effect did that have?

Describe your experience with health practitioners, medical doctors, nurses, hospital workers, alternative and complementary health practitioners and others who assisted you.

What were you told about your illness: diagnosis, symptoms, and prognosis for healing?

How were you treated? Describe what that person said or did.

How did you feel about the way you were treated?

Did you have a spiritual experience? Describe what happened.

How long has your illness lasted? Have you fully recovered yet?

What lingering effects are there in your body, mind, spirit, relationships?

How Have Your Health Practitioners Treated You?

Research shows that loving kindness, attention, warmth, touch, and belief in your ability to heal actually assist you in your healing process. Have your medical doctors or other health practitioners kept you waiting for very long periods of time? Have you been treated as a less important patient because you're affiliated with Managed Care, Medicaid, Medicare or other insurance that pays less than the doctor's preferred fees? Have you been examined carefully, tested adequately, listened to, and have all your questions been answered to your satisfaction? Is your doctor or health practitioner reachable by phone? How long does it take for you to schedule an appointment? Are you satisfied with the health care you have been given?

Your Healing History

Let's begin a life healing review, as far back as you can remember.

What has happened to your body, mind and spirit during your life?

What diseases, traumas, injuries and emotional hurts have you experienced?

What medications, shock treatments, surgeries or other professional medical or psychological treatments have you received?

What problems of yours were inherited, what was acquired, and how?

What have you done to cause your health problems, to make the symptoms worse or to alleviate symptoms and improve your health? What was the effect?

What have others -- health practitioners, friends, family, clergy -- done to cause your health problems, make the symptoms worse or to alleviate symptoms and improve your health? What was the effect?

How did you feel about yourself while you were ill?

How do you feel about yourself now, in relation to this illness?

What have been the long-term effects of your health problems and the way they were handled?

Your Healing Needs

Where in your life and body do you currently need healing?

How would you describe your current health, body image, and general emotional state?

How are your current relationships with friends, family, co-workers and lovers?

How is your financial situation, work, education, and career?

How do you spend your leisure time?

How comfortable is your current home?

How do you express yourself creatively?

Your Health Habits Inventory

List each of the following at the top of a page in your journal:

- *My Physical Health*
- *My Emotional and Mental Health*

Copyright © 2009, Revised 2023   *Heal Me … Please*   DrEricaGoodstone.com

- *My Social and Relationship Health*
- *My Sensual Health*
- *My Sexual Health*
- *My Spiritual* and *Intuitive Health*

Now, do take an inventory of the current state of your health: physical, emotional and mental, social and relationship, sensual, sexual; spiritual and intuitive. List words, phrases, sentences or entire descriptions in each category.

Change and Healing

Change and healing require faith and also conscious effort. If we continue to do what we've always done, we'll probably get what we've always gotten. As we age, we will experience diminishing returns on a poor health investment. **Let's do something different, do something positive for our own health - now!**

Your Health Investment Portfolio

In your journal draw a large circle. Divide the circle into parts, like the pieces of a pie.

O

Using different colored pencils, indicate the following:

What portion of my life do I devote to self-care?

What portion of my life do I devote to caring for others?

What portion of my life is filled with meaningful work and career?

What portion of my life is filled with basic chores and tasks?

What portion of my life is filled with leisure activities and play?

What portion of my life is devoted to rest, relaxation and rejuvenation?

What portion of your life is spent in meditation, prayer and spiritual practices?

Return on Your Health Investments

Maintaining good health represents a return on your investment.

What actions have your taken or not taken today and this week that are long-term investments in future ill health (unexpressed angry feelings, 3 cups of coffee for breakfast, procrastinating and worrying)

What actions have you taken today and this week that are positive self care habits and long-term investments in your future health (eating a well-balanced breakfast, remembering to breathe deeply, doing some aerobic exercise)?

YOUR COMMITMENT TO HEALING

Sit quietly, close your eyes and take a few long, slow, deep breaths. Read these the following questions a few times. Silently contemplate the meaning in your life. When you are ready, begin to write in your journal. Let your answers be as honest and thoughtful.

Remember, this is about your life, what you are willing to do to create the life you want.

Am I willing to end my commitment to suffering and begin my commitment to healing?

Copyright © 2009, Revised 2023   Heal Me ... Please   DrEricaGoodstone.com

Is my commitment to healing my life great enough to do whatever it takes to eliminate my own inner obstacles, fears and blocks?

Am I willing to accept the power of my mind to create, my heart's knowledge of truth, and the spiritual being that exists inside of me?

Am I willing to accept, with humility, my own smallness in comparison to the universal powers that exist?

What Does God Mean To You?

Open your eyes and begin to write - automatically - as the thoughts come to you. Do not stop to think or ponder or censure. Answer this simple question, *What does God mean to me?*

Following Your Own Spiritual Path

Sit comfortably. Take a few slow, deep and easy breaths. Imagine yourself as young child. In your mind, answer the following questions:

What did you believe about God and love, angels and spirits, mother, father, and life?

As you became more conscious, perhaps before you were able to form words, what did you know about spirits and spirituality?

What is your earliest memory about religion, spirituality and God?

With what religion were your mother, father or early caretakers raised?

What did your mother, father and earliest caretakers teach you, show you or believe themselves about God, church, religion and spirituality?

In your home was there a unified belief or divergent and conflictual beliefs?

Did God, angels, higher power, entities or anything otherworldly affect you as a young child?

Did you have a spiritual crisis at any point in your early years?

Did you ever turn away from God? If so, what caused this to happen?

What do you currently believe about God, religion, and spirituality?

What do you currently believe about reincarncation, psychic phenomena, ghosts, angels, entities, clairvoyance, witchcraft, spirits, spells, seances, energy transfers?

What religion or religious beliefs and concepts do you currently follow? Describe those beliefs.

What Does God Have To Do With Your Healing?

Young children are often quite spiritual. Children are likely to see, hear and claim to connect to spirits, angels and entities from other realms of existence. Some even appear to remember previous lives. Children who are abused, isolated or abandoned may retain their connection to this other world indefinitely. But as most of us become actively involved with friends, school, and social events, we tend to leave behind our earlier spiritual connections in favor of belonging and being accepted. Joining our parents' church or synagogue, we look there for our spirituality and redemption from pain and suffering. If we are lucky, our spiritual leaders are sincere, we feel connected to a higher power, and we learn to trust in life, ourselves, each other and in God.

Many of us are not so fortunate. Perhaps our parents or our pastors have instilled in us the fear of a wrathful, vindictive God. Perhaps our parents have taught us that God is a myth, does not exist, and that humans retain within themselves the ultimate power in life. Perhaps one of our parents believes in God while the other parent does not. Perhaps our parents follow different religions, each with entirely different beliefs, code of ethics, traditions and prescriptions for happiness.

Many of us experience a spiritual crisis, at a young age, that turns us away from God. For me, it was in my adolescence. Going to temple always reminded me of the early days with my father, who was deeply religious and internally spiritual. But my friends at the time were more interested in socializing and flirting with the boys. They did not share the sense of spiritual awe that I had always known. They did not seem to care about significance of the holy days or the power of prayer.

That day, I turned away from God, my religion, prayer and spirituality, for many years to come. Fortunately for me, my connection to God was eventually reawakened. My reawakening began with the consciousness raising groups of the 70's and 80's and intensive study of different spiritual and mystical traditions: Rosicrucians, Siddha Yoga, Kabbala, breathwork, and body therapies.

A weekend experience with my mentor, Ilana Rubenfeld, and my training in Rubenfeld Synergy and polarity therapy led me to my life's work, the complex and powerful integrative work known as body psychotherapy. For me, body psychotherapy brings together all the elements of a full life. Releasing whatever blocks us from experiencing the unity within our own body, mind and spirit, body psychotherapy helps us to open our hearts to love and be with others in meaningful relationships, and to feel our connection to a higher power or God.

Your Connection To God

Close your eyes. Take a few slow, easy, full breaths as you allow your body to relax.

Imagine that you have a direct connection to a higher source with the definite knowledge that you are safe, supported, and loved.

What if all you had to do in you life was to follow this higher guidance?

How would your life change?

Would you be more demanding or more forgiving of yourself and others?

Would you expect life to be a certain way or would you find wonder and acceptance in living life, the way it is, moment to moment?

Imagine living as if there is nothing you have to do, be, or become. Allow yourself to open your heart and mind to your own personal connection to all the knowledge that exists. Imagine that all answers will be provided for you if you ask and patiently wait to receive. Pause to examine your current life situation. Ask a question about what you want to change, improve, attain, or become. Sit quietly and listen for the answer.

The Joy of Suffering

Sometimes you choose to visit with a professional for help with a problem in our life. You may go to a physician and find you are not being seen for who you are, not listened to, and not really heard. You may go to a psychotherapist, speak what is true for you, and find that the therapist does not really understand you and perhaps offers advice you are not ready or willing to follow. You may choose to see an alternative and complementary practitioner who promises to offer what the traditional doctors could not. Once again, you may find you are not seen for who you are, not listened to, heard or understood.

Ultimately, you have to find a way to heal your own self. The joy in suffering is that your suffering, painful as it is, brings you closer to knowing your self. Nobody else can remove the stressors in your life, improve your diet, increase your exercise, get adequate sleep and rest, heal your thinking, balance your emotions, or forgive yourself for you. Each of us must find our own connection to God or something greater and beyond our own self.

Some religious groups believe that disease, illness and mental problems do not come from God and with proper thought alone, healing can and will occur.

Is your life exactly the way you always dreamed it could be? If the answer is "Yes," congratulations! Close the book now and continue enjoying your life. But if you're like the vast majority of us, even if your life is relatively good, in some ways you are not quite happy, not quite satisfied. Perhaps you're not happy with your work, your relationships, your appearance, your family, your friendships, or your health. Perhaps you seem to have everything you *should* want yet you find yourself sabatoging your good fortune, disappointing and hurting those closes to you.

Sometimes the most devastating events - death of a loved one, life-threatening illness, even complete mental breakdown - can be a gift for the healing of our soul. Unable to run and escape in our usual manner, we are forced to remain still, to face our true selves, reveal ourselves to the world, and to reconnect with our inner knowing.

The life we are currently living is not going to last, no matter what we do. The question is: How do you want to spend the limited time you have? What is your passion, your deepest desire, your life's purpose here on earth?

Are you currently fulfilling your life's goals, following your heart's desire?

If not, what are you waiting for?

LET ALL YOUR SENSES

SPEAK AS YOU HEAL

HEAL ME ... PLEASE

CHAPTER 2

LET ALL YOUR SENSES SPEAK

AS YOU HEAL

Touch Me Today

Touch me ... today
Feel me
With your hands
Hear me
With your heart
Speak to me
With your eyes
Love me
With your ears

Listen to
My silent voice
The one
That hasn't spoken
For a long time

Smell and taste
My memories
The ones I shared
With you
In some forgotten
Distant past

Allow your fingers
To explore
My inner being
Those secret places
That even I
Dare not go
Those held together
Tight spots
That lock the truth
Entombed
Inside of me

Touch me now
Let all our senses
Meet
Rejoice together
Now
As we explore
The depths
And heights
Of our connection
To each other
To life
To the source

Copyright © 9/20/97 Erica Goodstone, Ph.D.

Let Your Senses Speak To You

What Are Your Five Senses Revealing?

Every moment of every day we touch and are touched by all of our senses. View something our mind tells us is beautiful. Watch innocent children or carefree animals romp and play. Our mood may instantly change from gloomy, agitated or angry to peaceful and calm. Taste delicious food or sip a cool drink of water. Our mood may lift and we find we can somehow cope more easily with our problems. Sniff familiar and favorite scents, suddenly recalling people we have loved or earlier happy times. Our spirit may calm down in the moment. Hearing loving words can soothe away our physical aches and pains. Listening ears of one who cares may alleviate our longing for love, relive our sorrow, assuage our guilt and encourage us to persist in our struggles toward attaining our dreams.

Physical touch is the most powerful aphrodisiac in the world. Intentional loving touch heals. It heals our physical wounds, unbinds our psychological scars, and reminds us of our spiritual essence. Sensual touch makes all our sense come alive with new vitality. And intimate sexual touch can lead us to union with ourselves, our partner, and with God.

Physical touch is intimate. When we touch another person we discover who they are. When we are touched we cannot hide. Perceptive hands know all there is to know through touch.

You cannot know someone without touching them. You cannot touch someone without knowing them. You may choose not to consciously know what your body and mind sensed when you touched or were touched. And you can touch another person with any of your senses, not just physical touch.

If you believe words but do not believe your touch sensations, then you are favoring your sense of hearing. If you believe what you see but do not believe your touch sensations, you are favoring your sense of sight.

Your other two senses, taste and smell, are closely related to touch. We are all naturally attracted or repelled by the odor of another person's body. A person's state of physical and emotional health will affect the odor they emanate and the taste of their skin. The taste of another person can usually only be discovered in an intimate encounter.

So we have an order of intimacy from least intimate to most. Sight and sound and smell can be the least intimate. (A perfume or a body odor so strong that you smell it from a far distance; seeing someone who doesn't know you see them; overhearing a conversation not meant for your ears). Or these senses can be extremely intimate. E.g., a partner seductively undressing for your eyes only; whispers of sweet nothings directly into your ears; the scent of a special perfume that you love.

Touch and taste are always intimate. Recall the feeling of sitting too close or being touched in a private place by a stranger. Yet, all the senses are intimate. That's why we hide our head in shame (after a wrongdoing) or children hide behind mommy's skirt - not to be seen. Maybe we are afraid to speak or sing in front of large groups of people, or afraid to voice our opinions assertively - afraid to be listened to and heard. Americans often use deodorant or after-shave and cologne, afraid to allow another to smell us "au naturel". In many other countries, men and women to not attempt to cover up their natural bodily scents.

Of all the senses, taste is one we often share through tasting and sharing food together. However, most of us reserve the tasting of each other's bodily fluids to our sexual partners (and with the prevalence of disease to only a handful of select partners). And some of us choose not to share the intimacy of taste at all. Many abhor deep mouth kissing and refuse to engage in oral-genital contact. Many women are repulsed by the taste of a man's ejaculatory fluid. Many men dislike the taste or smell of a woman's vaginal fluids. Most of us would be repelled by fluids that emanate from the nose or ears or anus. Yet animals delight in sniffing and licking each other's entire bodies, anus and nostrils alike.

A developing fetus, still in its mother's womb, feels sensations, responds to sound and light, and becomes physiologically aroused. In fact, male fetuses have penile erections and female fetuses have vaginal lubrication, while still developing in the womb.

Reawakening Through Sensual Awareness

What is spiritual and sexual reawakening if not the exploration of our own bodily sensations and our inner voice and vision? We can begin by paying attention to all of our senses, one by one. Gradually increasing our sensual awareness through our eyes, ears, mouth, nose and skin will help us to become more receptive to the unique senses and scents of our most intimate partners. We will also find, in the still quiet of mindful attention, that we connect with something way beyond our own self, something infinite, powerful and the source of all that is or ever was.

WHAT DO YOU SEE?

OPEN YOUR EYES AND LOOK

Open your eyes wide and take a good look around you. Develop an artist's eye for detail.

Imagine wearing clear, neutral, objective, non-emotional glasses.

What do you see in your indoor environment every day?

> *Colors, shapes, patterns, arrangements, structure, cleanliness (or lack of).*
>
> *At home*
>
> *At work, school or leisure activity center*
>
> *At senior citizen center, prison, hospital, or other place you spend time at often*

What do you see in your outdoor environment every day?

> *Places, nature, stores, houses, buildings, destruction, construction*

What do you notice about people in your everyday life?

> *Physical appearance (beauty, height, weight, body shape, posture)*
>
> *Clothing (style, cost, color, fabrics, fit)*
>
> *Attitude, emotions, character traits, behavior*

Financial and professional status

Individuality, creativity or conformity

What do you notice about yourself?

Physical appearance (beauty, height, weight, body shape, posture)

Clothing (style, cost, color, fabrics, fit)

Attitude, emotions, character traits, behavior

Financial and professional status

Individuality, creativity or conformity

JUDGE WHAT YOUR EYES SEE

Imagine wearing dark, negative, judgmental glasses.

Critique and criticize what you see in your indoor environment every day.

Colors, shapes, patterns, arrangements, structure, cleanliness (or lack of).

At home

At work, school or leisure activity center

At senior citizen center, prison, hospital, or other place you spend time at often

Critique and criticize what you see in your outdoor environment every day.

Places, nature, stores, houses, buildings, destruction, construction

Critique and criticize the people you see in your everyday life.

Physical appearance (beauty, height, weight, body shape, posture0

    Clothing (style, cost, color, fabrics, fit)

    Attitude, emotions, character traits, behavior

    Financial and professional status

    Individuality, creativity or conformity

What do you notice about yourself?

    Physical appearance (beauty, height, weight, body shape, posture)

    Clothing (style, cost, color, fabrics, fit)

    Attitude, emotions, character traits, behavior

    Financial and professional status

    Individuality, creativity or conformity

Imagine wearing rose colored, positive, loving and unconditionally accepting glasses.

Praise and enjoy what you see in your indoor environment every day.

    Colors, shapes, patterns, arrangements, structure, cleanliness (or lack of).

    At home

    At work, school or leisure activity center

At senior citizen center, prison, hospital, or other place you spend time at often.

Praise and enjoy what you see in your outdoor environment every day.

Places, nature, stores, houses, buildings, destruction, construction

Praise and enjoy the people you see in your everyday life.

Physical appearance (beauty, height, weight, body shape, posture0

Clothing (style, cost, color, fabrics, fit)

Attitude, emotions, character **traits**, *behavior*

Financial and professional status

Individuality, creativity or conformity

What do you notice about yourself?

Physical appearance (beauty, height, weight, body shape, posture)

Clothing (style, cost, color, fabrics, fit)

Attitude, emotions, character traits, behavior

Financial and professional status

Individuality, creativity or conformity

SET YOUR SIGHTS

Close your eyes.

Imagine a present scene, a picture of your world the way it is right now.

    Your Environment

    People

    Yourself

See beneath the surface.

    See beyond people's egos, defenses, fears, separating actions

    See beyond your own ego, defenses, fears, separating actions

    See your dreams, your potential, your capabilities

Imagine living in your ideal world.

    Describe your indoor and outdoor environments.

    Describe the people in your life.

    Describe yourself.

Imagine a future scene, as if it were occurring right now.

    Your environment is clean, exciting, peaceful, and everything you want it to be.

    People are loving, accepting, beautiful, and everything you want them to be.

Copyright © 2009, Revised 2023   *Heal Me … Please*   DrEricaGoodstone.com

You are loving, accepting, beautiful, and everything you want to be.

Now, hold a vision of your present world, the way it is right now

And at the same time…

Hold a vision of your ideal world, the way you would like it to be in your future.

Hold these two visions simultaneously for 30 seconds.

Then let the visions go, open your eyes, and go for a walk for a few minutes. Do this every day, preferably morning and evening. Watch miracles happen!

DO YOU HEAR WHAT I HEAR?

Many of us often do not really listen. Our ears are hearing but our minds are busy calculating and interpreting, sometimes even before the speaker has begun talking. I call this defensive listening. You are listening with a closed mind, perhaps to protect your mind, to protect your genitals, to protect your heart, or even to protect your most valued spiritual beliefs.

OPEN YOUR EARS AND LISTEN

What sounds do you hear in the background?

What sounds irritate or annoy you?

What sounds or music make your smile and feel warm all over?

How Do You Listen To Yourself?

What bodily sensations do you pay attention to and what do you, ignore?

How do you respond to what you hear?

> *Brace yourself, hold it all together, stand up to, stand my ground, dig my heels in,*
>
> *Keep a stiff upper lip, lift my spirits, put up a good front,*
>
> *Get my back up against the wall, keep a smile on my face, reach out, hold it in?*

How Do You Listen To Others?

Do you hear what you want to hear and ignore the rest?

Copyright © 2009, Revised 2023   *Heal Me ... Please*   DrEricaGoodstone.com

Do you listen to the words and the nuances of meanings?

Do you listen to the nonverbal messages - body language and facial expressions?

Do you listen to the tone, attitude, pitch, and quality of voice?

Do you consider who is speaking, the source of the words you hear - the speaker's background, experience, prejudices and perspectives)?

Do you pay attention to you own bodily feelings as you listen to the words of others?

Who Do You Hear When You Listen?

Do you hear your mother, father, sister, brother, aunt, uncle, grandmother, grandfather, teacher, minister, school bully...?

Do you hear someone who is about to tease you, abuse you, ignore you, humiliate you, appreciate you, play with you, love you....?

Do you listen for acceptance, love, rejection, approval, safety, denial, disrespect, disregard, judgement, criticism, praise, insult, abandonment?

Do you expect to hear intellectual content, emotional understanding, criticism, sarcasm, drama, or worldly wisdom?

Do you feel heard, understood and connected or ignored, put down and alone?

How do you think, feel and respond when you hear what you are expecting to hear?

How do you think, feel and respond when you don't hear what you expect to hear?

What Are Your Listening and Speaking Goals?

My listening and speaking goals are to

- connect to my truth, what is true for me, in every moment of my life.
- listen and respond to the wisdom of my body and all my senses.
- respond to the world and the people in it from my own truth.

What Are Your Listening and Speaking Goals?

What Do You Want To Say … And To Whom?

Copyright © 2009, Revised 2023   *Heal Me … Please*   DrEricaGoodstone.com

Allow your beliefs to live, breathe, and to change form as life shows you another way. **Don't sell yourself short.** Each of us is unique and has our unique logic, beauty and wisdom. Maybe you've been put down, criticized, or judged and you believe you are less valuable and know less than others. You probably have much sharper antennae to recognize signs of impending abuse. You may know more about how to leave your body, to dissociate, so that you do not have to feel the full effect of the pain. You may know more about how to compulsively complete a task regardless of how your body feels.

We can help each other. None of us sees the whole picture. Even the most enlightened Guru is not living your life, with your friends, your parents, your lovers, or your spouse. The enlightened Guru meditates and chants in an environment surrounded by devotees and followers.

I often wonder what would happen to the Guru's perfect sublime state if he or she lived with your parents or spouse and was in close contact with your friends. Would the Guru maintain that state of calm and peace and wisdom and transform everyone else? Or would this enlightened master become frustrated, angry, agitated, without the time, space and clear energy to meditate.

I remember Hilda Charlton, an enlightened master in New York, could no longer be around beginners' energy. Another well-known guru stopped having darshan with beginning followers because of a back problem. Another wonderful, enlightened meditation group was unable to remain in New York City because of the intense negative energy they felt.

We are all human beings with bodies that utilized our five senses. We all need to listen to each other and especially, to listen to our own self.

OPEN YOUR SENSE OF SMELL

BREATHING

Sit quietly and close your eyes.

Keep your mouth closed, lips touching, teeth apart inside your mouth.

Breathe slowly, softly and easily through your nose 10X.

Breathe through your left nostril.

> *Squeeze your right nostril closed with your right thumb.*
>
> *Inhale and exhale through your left nostril 10X.*
>
> *Remove your right thumb and rest.*

How do you feel?

Did you feel any difference breathing through only one nostril?

Breathe through your right nostril.

Squeeze your left nostril closed with your left thumb.

Inhale and exhale through your right nostril 10X

Remove your left thumb and rest.

How do you feel now?

Did you notice any difference, breathing through your right or left nostril?

Breathe through both nostrils 10X.

How do you feel?

Did you notice any difference, breathing through both nostrils?

Alternative breathing through right and left nostrils.

Place your right thumb against your right nostril.

Place your left thumb against your left nostril.

Squeeze your right nostril closed as you inhale and exhale through your left.

Squeeze your left nostril closed as you inhale and exhale through your right.

Continue alternating until you have completed 5 rounds on each side.

SMELLING

Take a smelling tour of your kitchen.

Begin in the cabinets.

    Open the jars or cans and smell the different spices, sauces, condiments, beverages, cereals, crackers, vitamins, herbs, other foods.

Open the refrigerator.

    Open the jars and packages and smell the different fruits, vegetables, dairy, juices, leftovers, beer, soda, meats or meat substitutes.

Take a smelling tour of your bathroom. Yes, even if it has a malodorous residue.

    Open the jars and tubes.

    Smell the various oils, creams, lotions, soaps, toothpaste, detergents, medications.

Take a smelling tour of your closet.

    Smell your dirty laundry.

    Smell your freshly cleaned clothing, still hanging with the cleaner's tags or recently removed from the washer and dryer..

Smell your body.

Scan through your body.

Notice the different scents and odors emanating from different parts of your own body.

Take a walk into town.

Before you leave, pay attention to the scent of your own apartment or house.

Intentionally walk past coffee houses, bakeries, fish markets, meat markets or different sections of your local supermarket.

Find the bath, cosmetics, and drug departments.

Go to a linen shop and a clothing store.

Consciously smell the variety of scents and odors.

When you return home, notice the immediate impact of the scent in your apartment or home.

OPEN YOUR SENSE OF TASTE

Taste Your World

Take a tasting tour of your kitchen.

Begin in the cabinets.

    Open some boxes, jars or cans and taste different spices, sauces, condiments, crackers, cereals, other foods.

Open the refrigerator.

    Open the jars and packages and smell the different fruits, vegetables, dairy, juices, leftovers, beer, soda, meats or meat substitutes.

    Take a tiny taste of a wide variety of different foods and condiments.

Taste yourself.

    Taste your fingers, wrists, forearms, knees, ankles, palms, hair - whatever bodyparts you are able to reach and feel safe enough to taste.

Take a walk into town.

Before you leave, recall the tastes available in your own apartment or house.

Intentionally walk past restaurants, coffee houses, bakeries, fish markets, meat markets, different sections of your local supermarket.

Intentionally taste foods of many different types, shapes, colors textures and drink a variety of different beverages.

When you return home, compare the outside tastes to those available in your apartment or home.

Spend an entire month consciously tasting as many different foods and drink as many different beverages as you can.

Keep a running list of every type of food and drink you have tried - and your sensual reactions.

OPEN YOUR SENSE OF TOUCH

TOUCH YOUR WORLD

How do you feel about touching yourself?

How do you feel about touching others? Who? Why?

How do you feel about others touching themselves?

How do you feel about others touching you? Who? Why?

Touch your own hands.

> *Feel the texture, warmth, quality, roughness, smoothness, energy*
>
> *As if your right hand and left hands are two different people*
>
>> 1. *Which is male, which is female?*
>>
>> 2. *Which is aggressive, which is more passive?*
>>
>> 3. *Which is parent, which is child?*
>>
>> 4. *Which is playful, which is serious?*
>>
>> 5. *Which feels good, hurts?*
>
> *Caress each hand with your other hand, with your lips, your teeth*

Touch as many different parts of your body that you feel safe and comfortable touching.

Touch some body parts that you usually would avoid touching.

Take a touching tour of your kitchen.

Begin in the cabinets.

> *Open the jars or cans and touch the different spices, sauces, condiments, beverages, cereals, crackers, vitamins, herbs, other foods.*

Open the refrigerator.

Copyright © 2009, Revised 2023 *Heal Me ... Please* DrEricaGoodstone.com

Open the jars and packages and touch the different fruits, vegetables, dairy, juices, leftovers, beer, soda, meats or meat substitutes.

Take a touching tour of your bathroom.

Open the jars and tubes.

Touch the various bottles, oils, creams, lotions, soaps, toothpaste, detergents, medications.

Take a touching tour of your closets and drawers..

Touch the different fabrics, textures, shapes, materials.

Touch the hangers and cleaners cellophane wrapping.

Take a walk into a nearby town.

Intentionally walk past different stores: coffee houses, bakeries, fish markets, meat markets, different sections of your local supermarket. Find the bath, cosmetics, and drug departments.

Go to a linen shop and different clothing stores. Feel the quality of the different materials, scarves, hats, gloves, shoes, socks, panties, bras, belts, handbags, suits, shirts, blouses, sweaters, furs

Go to a bedding store. Lie down on different mattresses. Compare the effect of hard and soft mattresses, feather and polyurethane pillows.

Copyright © 2009, Revised 2023   Heal Me ... Please   DrEricaGoodstone.com

Go to a hardware store, a picture framing store, a novelty store.

Feel the various textures, shapes and qualities of the store's items.

The questions and exercises in this chapter were designed to help you expand your sensual awareness and responsiveness. If you have completed all the exercises, you have also learned how to tune into your own body and allow your body's wisdom to speak to you. As you continue to increase your own sensual awareness, you expand your healing potential exponentially and you also become more readily attuned to the unique sensual responsiveness of everyone, including and especially, your most intimate partner/s.

TOUCHING STORIES

HEALING THROUGH TOUCH

AND

BODY PSYCHOTHERAPY

HEAL ME ... PLEASE

CHAPTER 3

TOUCHING STORIES

Healing Through Touch

And Body Psychotherapy

The Story of My Life

The story of my life
Unfolds
In your presence
Private burdens
Shameful secrets
Held within my lonely
Heart
Come pouring out
I cry
I laugh

I kick and scream
You understand
You know the price
Of long held pain
The half-lived life
In fear
In shame
I let you see me
As I am
No judge
No jury
No pretense or sham
You make it safe
For me to be
As I slowly open
Becoming free.

Copyright © 8/20/99 Erica Goodstone, Ph.D.

Touching Stories

In this chapter, we explore the healing potential of body psychotherapy through stories of real people's lives. These stories are excerpts of actual case histories, therapy sessions, emotional responses, and eventual healing that took place in my office. Names and identifying personal characteristics have been altered to protect anonymity. None of my clients will be able to say with certainty, "That's me!" Yet, as we read these stories, each of us may recognize something familiar within ourselves.

As you read this chapter, ask yourself the following questions:

About The Stories:

How do I feel about this person, situation, or emotion?

Does anything about this story feel familiar or cause me to feel uneasy, anxious, angry, or sad?

About Body Psychotherapy:

Is this something I could use?

What would happen if I freely expressed my emotions and paid attention to my bodily sensations?

What would happen if I was willing to face the truth about my own life?

George's Handshake

George walked into my office, sat in his chair and immediately said, *"I'm not sure if I should be here, if this is what I need, if I even need therapy."* Describing his marriage as better than ever, he insisted, *"I love my wife. Sex with her is wonderful. It's just that ... well ... I look at women everywhere. I get turned on and even masturbate thinking about other women. Sometimes I go for massages ... you know ... the sensual ones. Lately I've been hanging out at topless bars - not the seedy kind. These are high class places, of course."*

Throughout the session, George's statements sounded believable until, as he was leaving, he shook my hand. **His handshake said it all!** I had the sense that he was not really there. Given his body size and structure - tall, lean and muscular - I would have expected a strong, solid handshake. But when I shook his hand, I felt as if there was nothing there to hold onto. Not completely limp, it was just hardly there.

George's body holds the key to understanding his insatiable desire for variety and new sexual stimulation. Not being conscious and actually suppressing his own internal sensations, he has difficulty connecting openly with others.

Being intimate with another person, physical and emotional as well as sensual and sexual, requires that we accept our own totality, including limitations and insecurities. It is not necessary to live a life of quiet shame and discontent or disdainful superiority, thinking we are less valuable or more worthy than others. We do not need to keep others from seeing our imperfections. We do not need others to be our own ideal of perfection.

When we are touched in a sensitive, healing way, communicating to us that we are seen, heard, understood, and okay as we are, miraculous changes occur. Our problems take a back seat to a sense of connectedness to all of humanity. We discover how powerful we really are and how much we affect others peoples' lives every day.

Lana's Unconsummated Marriage

At her first counseling session, Lana explained, *"I never enjoyed sex …even before I met my husband. If he left me alone, I'd be perfectly content to never do it."*

Her history revealed a painful, traumatic upbringing with a cold and often sadistic mother who had shown disgust with Lana's bodily functions, a gentle but unavailable workaholic father, and an older brother who sexually molested her over many years. It became Lana's lifelong quest to prove that she was beautiful and clean enough to be loved. Years of talk therapy and the pursuit by numbers of men, could not erase her deep-seated belief that she was unclean, ugly, and unworthy of love.

Although she loved her husband and knew he was a good man, extremely kind, patient, and nothing like her abusive brother, she just couldn't allow herself to feel pleasure when he touched her. Her mother's disgust and disapproval remained palpably locked inside her body, along with the painful memories of her brother's unwanted advances.

The pain and sadness of Lana's early touch memories prevented her from being able to enjoy pleasurable sexuality with her loving husband. As her body was re-touched in a healing way, she allowed herself to express her deepest emotions and her body posture became noticeably more relaxed. Eventually, over time, Lana actually began to feel desire and sexual pleasure with her husband.

Having intimate physical and emotional contact with another person, requires self-acceptance and emotional freedom. We forgive those who have caused us pain and we forgive our self for our weaknesses, insecurities, and self-indulgences. We no longer expect our self to be perfect to please others.

The Revitalization of Steven's Life

As Steven entered my office, I noticed his breathing was shallow and the movement in his neck and shoulders was limited. His symptoms included high blood pressure, severe anxiety, and difficulty sleeping. Without much emotion, Steven explained his predicament, *"I've been at the same job for over 10 years. They're downsizing, piling more and more work on the people who are still here. I can't afford to quit, but I'm miserable going to work. I take medication to lower my blood pressure and lately I have trouble sleeping. I've been with my girlfriend Paula for years, too long. I think I want to break up, but I can't make up my mind. Lately we've been fighting a lot. She's bothers me with her doubts and insecurities which makes me feel more anxious. And she complains I don't listen to her."*

During the first few sessions, Steven alternately complained about his job and about his relationship with Paula. In the third session, as he pounded his fist into a pillow and yelled at his girlfriend as if she was present in the room, something different happened. He screamed, *"You selfish bitch. You don't stop complaining about your problems. What about me?"* Suddenly he stopped! Tears filled his eyes.

In that moment he realized these were his father's exact words. He realized he was repeating his father's pattern with his mother. An imaginary dialogue with his girlfriend, in my office, enabled him to realize that he had been repeating a family pattern. He now wanted to change the negative way he had been treating and responding to Paula.

After a few more body therapy sessions, Steven's breathing was becoming apparently fuller and easier.. In his seventh session he told me, *"I'm sleeping better at night. I even took a few days off from work. Now it doesn't seem so bad to be there."* In that session, I worked to release the tension in his neck and shoulders, encouraging him to move his neck into the yoga fish position, lying on his back with the top of his head on the body therapy table and his chin pointed up in the air.

At first, he complained that this was an impossible maneuver. But over the next few weeks, he was able to actually move his head and neck separately from his shoulders. A few weeks later he told me, *"I feel like a new man. I never knew I could move like that."*

As his habitual bodily tensions lessened, Steven's energy level and creativity increased. He showed me an article he had recently submitted to a few magazines for possible publication. At the same time he expressed a renewed sense of passion and desire for his girlfriend. For the first time since the very beginning of their relationship, he was taking Paula on a vacation to a tropical island resort.

The Truth About John

When John enters a room, it is difficult not to notice him. Over 6 feet tall, with broad shoulders, a well-developed muscular body, and a warm, engaging smile, he would appear to be highly appealing to woman. However, by the time he arrived in my office at age 33, he had dated only a few women in his entire life and had never attempted any sexual contact beyond a simple kiss and only the briefest of hugs. During his first date with a woman, he would tell her he was afraid of sex and being close. Rarely did his relationships last beyond a second or third date. Although he claimed to have a few close male friends, he did not share his inner thoughts or true feelings with anyone. Afraid of letting others know how insecure he really was, he walked around with a chip on his shoulder, easily angered into violent behavior. As a young child he had been abused by older boys in the neighborhood, humiliated by teachers about his poor study habits, and teased by his family about his shyness around girls.

John's work in therapy involved letting go of his pretenses and letting down his guard. It took quite a while before John stopped censoring every thought to make sure it was acceptable. He needed to be reassured over and over that it was safe for him to express his thoughts and feelings in the moment. At one point, he admitted a lifelong fear he had that he might be gay. John's major overhaul came when he recovered his childhood sense of shame at not being "man enough" to defend himself against all the people who had humiliated and abused him. He also expressed some anger toward his parents, his mother for not protecting him and his father for not being a strong masculine figure in his life.

As John's familiar armored posture and frozen smile gradually softened, he began to feel vulnerable, exposed and more frightened out in the world. His familiar defenses, relying on his muscular physique, distancing himself, or playing the victim, no longer shielded him from his own painful feelings. It took a long time, several years of exploring his life issues and feeling his underlying emotions, before John was able to finally feel safe in the world. For a while, he needed almost daily reassurance that he would survive the demise of his defenses and be able to enjoy life being himself. Eventually he overcame his fear of connection and began to date women – and enjoy it.

Carol's Vagina Speaks

Carol, an attractive woman in her early thirties, began by telling me, "I never really enjoyed the sexual act, but I wanted a boyfriend and I knew men wanted sex. So I guess I just did it to please them." She explained, "We were always in a hurry. His parents were about to come home or we were in the car and somebody might see us if we lingered too long. So I guess I was never very stimulated or turned on."

In one session, Carol talked about the pain she had always felt in her vagina. I asked her to imagine what this body might say if it had a voice and could speak. After some initial hesitation, these words emerged from Carol, "Why did you ignore me? Didn't you know I hurt? I needed you to pay attention to me, to treat me gently."

As we explored further, we discovered that Carol came from a long line of highly educated, intellectual women who valued their brains and devalued their bodies. Despising femininity, the women in Carol's family were not proud of the body parts that distinguished them as female.

Carol's lifelong sexual problem could not be treated with medication, counseling, or even traditional sex therapy. It was not mechanical stimulation, external lubrication, or behavior modification that was needed. Internal dialogue, gentle, caring touch, and reconnection to the sensations in her body helped Carol to recover pleasurable feelings.

Lifelong shame about her intimate body parts gave way to an appreciation of her female body. As Carol learned to accept and love her own body, she began to enjoy and even crave the attention she received from men. Her body responded with heightened sexual desire. As a result, she dressed more stylishly, no longer hiding the natural curves of her body. To her surprise and delight, she received more male attention than ever before and more invitations to go out on dates than she could handle.

Louis' Panic Attacks

Louis, a part-time student in his late twenties, had experienced panic attacks all his life, but previously only in really frightening situations like speaking in front of his class or taking an important exam. *"Now the panic is occurring more often,"* he said. *"Lately I feel panicked when I walk into my office building, when I get on public transportation, even while I'm standing on line at a supermarket. There are beautiful women everywhere. If I look at a woman and she looks back at me, my body freezes. I feel as though I will pass out. I try to get out of there as fast as I can. By the time I'm outside, I can hardly breathe. Can you help me?"*

With Louis, the immediate task was to expand and increase his natural breathing pattern to lessen the possibility of another panic attack. Together, we observed the way he was holding his body in a state of defensive alertness, barely inhaling and exhaling, as if he is perpetually preparing to attack or be attacked. Through gentle touch, he was encouraged to progressively relax his body, part by part.

After many months of sessions, one day Louis spontaneously curled into a fetal position and began rocking. When I placed a hand lightly on his back, he began to whimper. Tears came, followed by deep, full belly sobbing. When he finally quieted down, his body appeared more relaxed than I had ever seen it before. For the first time in our work together, he was breathing deeply, inhaling and exhaling fully. When he sat up, a shy smile crossed his face. All he could say was, *"Thank you."*

Louis' panic attacks gradually diminished. Now, whenever he felt a panic coming on, he turned inward, observing which part of his body was tense. At the moment when he felt most afraid, Louis would inhale deeply and exhale slowly, allowing his body tension to naturally dissipate.

As he gained control over his breathing, Louis was finally ready to talk about the painful childhood experiences that had kept his body "on guard" for life. Raised by a controlling and angry father and a mother who played a traditionally submissive housewife role, Louis admitted he had not cried since he was very young, when his father beat him with a strap if he did not behave "like a man". For Louis, not behaving like a man was humiliating. But behaving like a man was also terrifying since his father had not taught him how. **It was the breath of life that saved Louis.** As he breathed more easily, he became less fearful of life and more comfortable in the presence of women.

Henry's Tears

Henry, a silver-haired stately businessman in his mid-fifties, took immediate control of the situation. He informed me that he had no time to waste. Looking over at the bodywork table he asked, *"How do I get from here,"* pointing to his less than functioning groin, *"to there?"* indicating the future, free from sexual impotence. *"I've already tried Viagra,"* he said. *"It worked all right for awhile. But I never needed to take anything before. I don't want to be dependent on a drug for the rest of my life."* He explained that he was curious about the way I work, but really doubted that allowing his body to be manipulated and feeling his feelings was going to cause his erection problem to disappear.

Henry described his marriage of many years. *"I love my wife so much. Denise is the best. She's beautiful and so intelligent. We have two great kids. I have a great life. Sex with my wife has always been wonderful. Sometimes I would come home in the middle of the day just to be with her. She was always hot and ready for me. I don't want to be with anybody else and I don't want to push her away. But lately I don't know what's happening. I get started, things seem great, and then poof. It goes down and won't come back. I'm scared. My wife tells me not to worry, but I'm sure she's been wondering what's wrong with me. I was at my wit's end when I took Viagra for the first time. Luckily it worked. But I never did tell Denise about it. I don't know what to do."*

Henry decided to go for it and signed up for a series of sessions. Many men in his position, afraid of losing their potency, might choose instead to turn to massage parlors, hookers, pornography, phone sex, and online relationships for sexual reassurance. But they are living precariously. If their private sexual activities are discovered, their unsuspecting, betrayed partners may respond strongly and even choose to end the relationship.

During the history session, Henry described a rather idyllic childhood. His parents were deeply in love, expressing affection and sexual desire for each other openly. He grew up close to his younger sister, with lots of friends and even girlfriends from the earliest age he could remember. His sister and he had been given every advantage, from attending Ivy League universities to socializing with an elite crowd.

Then Henry talked about Lucy, his high school sweetheart, his first love. Having shared wonderful, loving and exciting times together, they had planned to marry as soon as he graduated from college. Henry's father believed that Lucy, from a working class family, would not be an asset to his upper class, cultured lifestyle. When Henry went away to college, his father contacted Lucy to tell her it would be best for all concerned if she stopped seeing his son. Brokenhearted but still hopeful, she had called Henry to discuss the matter. Not paying much attention, he brushed her off with a sarcastic comment. Believing, erroneously, that Henry agreed with his father and would eventually break up with her, she decided to be the one to end the relationship first.

When she told Henry she no longer wanted to see him, he did not pursue her. He just let her go. That was the first and last time Henry remembered crying, except once in his early childhood when he had come running to mommy for comfort and she had scolded him, saying that boys must be strong.

Stopping to clear his throat and showing his obvious annoyance, he said to me,

"I don't understand what any of this has to do with losing my erections now. That happened when I was 18. I'm 54 now and I haven't thought about Lucy in years. I've been with Denise all my adult life and we love each other. Our sex life has always been wonderful."

A little more probing, however, revealed that his wife, Denise, was quite a perfectionist and liked her life to remain in perfect order. Henry had enjoyed complying with Denise's demands, convinced that it kept him on his toes and fueled his continual passion for his wife. On top of the world for over twenty years, his businesses had been flourishing and expanding. Lately, however, business was slowing down, and for the first time he had to downsize. Instead of using his creative talents toward establishing new business ventures, he now had to close some offices and fire a few trusted employees. A few sessions later, as he relaxed on the body therapy table, a tear appeared in the corner of his right eye. The realization came to him, *"All my life I've been in control. I chose the college I wanted. I got almost straight A's. I married the most beautiful woman and my children grew up exactly as I would have wanted. I had control of all my businesses and it felt as if nothing could stop me - until now. Everything is changing. I have to curtail my businesses and I could lose a substantial amount of money. I'm terrified of telling Denise. This is the second time in my whole life I remember feeling such fear and a sense of impending doom. The last time this happened was when I was away at college and Lucy told me on the phone that she had to stop dating me, that she was seeing someone else, and that she no longer loved me. I couldn't believe my ears. My body went numb. I felt a knot in my stomach.* **That's when the tears came!** *My roommate asked me what was wrong. For a few minutes I was unable to speak and then my heart literally closed up. I never cried again! A few years later I met Denise, took her on a whirlwind of exciting dates and never let her get off the whirlwind until now. I'm afraid if I don't keep her life exciting and busy and passionately sexual, she will suddenly leave me just as Lucy did, so many years ago."*

Henry's insight transformed his marriage. He began to tell his wife the truth about his declining businesses and his fear of her deserting him if times got bad. He even brought her with him to therapy to improve the way they communicate with each other.

After years of hiding his emotions and striving to please his critical, demanding mother first, and then his equally critical wife, he finally discovered the joy of letting himself feel and express his real feelings. After years of marriage, Henry had finally revealed the sensitive, not so strong, even vulnerable and frightened side of himself. Much to his surprise, his usually critical and demanding wife did not desert him. Instead, she actually touched him more tenderly than he had ever remembered. Realizing his marriage was on solid ground, no matter what happened to his finances, his erections naturally returned to normal. Their sex life took on a new, more sensual and romantic style.

Henry's emotions were his ally. Without the anxiety, fear and breaking down into tearful sadness, Henry stood to lose everything dear to him, his wife, his self-respect, and his wonderful family life.

What Is Body Psychotherapy?

Body psychotherapy is a life transforming, therapeutic experience. The counseling is similar to psychotherapy that is not focused on the body and does not involve touch. But when our bodies are touched as we are talking about our life issues, there is a powerful synergistic effect. Even very gentle touch re-connects us with memories of sensations and emotions stored within our body tissues. Unexpectedly, we might find ourselves crying, yelling, or even laughing uncontrollably. As we feel emotions we haven't felt in a long time, we may have a life-changing realization.

Professional certification and licensing boards have specific guidelines and strict ethical codes for the practice of body psychotherapy. Before receiving any sessions, we are entitled to be told what to expect during a session. The therapist must have our agreement before engaging in any verbal dialogue, touch, or other therapeutic processes. If we feel uncomfortable at any point, it is important to immediately inform the therapist. Remember, we always have the right to say, "No." We must trust our own reactions and responses. Nobody is a more qualified expert on how we feel in any given moment. Healing happens most easily when we feel safe, respected and heard.

The common element of all body psychotherapy methods is the use of touch. Touch is used differently and for different purposes within the various modalities. Some body psychotherapists (Bioenergetic analysts, Reichian therapists, Core Energetic therapists, Radix practitioners) may at times use forceful, deep, even painful pressure, in an attempt to break through bodily armoring and emotional resistance. Organismic body psychotherapists sometimes actually use their own physical bodies to touch and support their clients to let go of habitual tension patterns. Other body psychotherapists (Hakomi, Focusing, Rosen Method, Integrative Body Psychotherapy, Rubenfeld Synergy therapists) utilize guided imagery, gentle touch and even touch that is off the body in the energetic field. If one style of body psychotherapy does not feel right, for any reason, choose a different therapist whose style of working feels more comfortable.

For me, body psychotherapy is gentle and always respectful of the client. Although my certification and the framework for my sessions is Rubenfeld Synergy, Somatoemotional Release and Polarity Therapy, I have incorporated many techniques from other counseling, body therapy, and body psychotherapy modalities. It is like having a bag of tricks at my fingertips, literally.

How Does the Body Psychotherapy Process Work?

Our body does not lie. The way we hold and move our body is the key to understanding ourself and reaching our full human potential. When we recognize and express our deepest feelings, the cells in our body respond accordingly. Our tissues soften, our posture lengthens and widens, and we view our world with greater clarity.

In body psychotherapy, both therapist and client are on a sacred healing journey together. We not only touch each other, we also explore together the deeper psychological, symbolic and interpersonal meanings in our life. When we are touched, we are no longer the person we pretend to be, want to be, or perceive our self to be. Feelings sometimes intensify, but over time the intensity gradually diminishes. We build a solid base of self-awareness, self-acceptance, and self-love.

Body psychotherapy is about life, your life, my life, and our lives together on this earth. Being willing to feel and express our raw emotions, we have the rare opportunity to release the pain and anguish inherent in the human condition. We can actually live the remainder of our lives in a state of peaceful joy, more readily willing to acknowledge, accept, and love our most intimate partners.

Body Psychotherapy Energizes Our Brain

Touch enhances our body awareness and assists us to relax. Our brains receive, interpret, and transmit to our bodies the information received by our senses. Chemicals in the form of neurotransmitters travel along pathways of the brain searching for a home in specific neuroreceptors, located within our brain and throughout our body. Our circulation improves, our breathing increases, our posture re-aligns, our face softens, our voice deepens, and our internal organs function with less restriction. Energy flows within our own bodies and also flows outward, connecting us in unseen ways with people, animals, plants and even nonliving objects. Our energy flow can be blocked, stimulated, drained, sedated or even depleted. Our "electromagnetic field" has been measured and documented through Kirlian photography. Asian healing methods track this "chi" energy through the "meridians" (energy channels) in our body. Yogis have observed this "kundalini" energy traveling upward through the "nadis" (small energy pathways) to the "chakras" (energy centers). As we are touched in body psychotherapy, our energy flows more freely within our own body and outward to the world around us.

Body Psychotherapy Allows us to Breathe in Life

Breath is life. When we breathe our first breath, we are alive. When we gasp our final breath, we are no longer alive. Many of us are living every day in an almost "near death" state. Although we are breathing enough to remain alive, we are not breathing enough to feel. Restricting our breathing restricts our life. We hold our breath to hold in our emotions. We hold our breath to not feel pain. But when we don't allow ourselves to feel pain, we also do not feel pleasure and joy. **Body psychotherapy helps us to regain the fullness of our breath and the fullness of our life.**

Body Psychotherapy Reveals and Uncovers Our Truth

Truth heals - when realized, acknowledged, and accepted. Every bodily sensation mirrors our thoughts, emotions, desires and disappointments. Through conscious awareness of our these sensations, moment to moment, we discover what is true for us. As we face and admit our personal truth, the path is finally clear for our pain and sorrow to dissolve. We recognize our responsibility to thrive in this life, to shine our own light brightly for ourselves and for others who may be hiding in the dark. **Body psychotherapy helps us to know our own self as we remove the armoring that hides the truth of our being from our own consciousness.**

Body Psychotherapy Helps Us to Heal

In body psychotherapy, memories of our past experiences emerge into our current awareness. We scrutinize the details of each crucial segment of our life until this piece gradually recedes into the background, merging into the core of our being. New pieces emerge into our awareness and the process continues. Rough edges of our personality reveal themselves and slowly dissolve as we examine the hidden meanings. We become exhibitionists, revealing our most intimate and shameful secrets to another human being. We become voyeurs of our own life. We watch our responses as our fears, thoughts, desires, compulsions, and not so acceptable emotions, are exposed. The long, slow process of healing begins as we bring our demons into the light, shine our mental flashlight on our problems, and forgive our self and others for being human. **As we heal through body psychotherapy we are able to integrate positive and negative aspects of our self and the world in which we live.**

Body Psychotherapy Reopens Our Heart to Love

Emotions are natural human gifts, revealing our innermost desires. We respond emotionally to our own internal sensations and to the physical and emotional states of people around us. With intensely painful stimulation that we cannot eliminate or control, we adapt by closing off our emotions and closing our hearts. Sharing heart talk, honest emotional responses, while being gently touched by an accepting and caring therapist, we allow our self to experience the full range of our emotions. **Body psychotherapy assists us to feel our emotions as we heal our bruised or broken hearts.**

Body Psychotherapy Reawakens Our Sensual, Sexual and Spiritual Aliveness

Our sexual problem can be the gift that sets us free. Our body provides us with all sorts of messages reminding us to slow down, rest, change our habits, speak up, run away, hide, nurture ourselves, or to seek help. When we pay attention to the sensational world around us and inside of us, we see beautiful colors, hear pleasing sounds, smell fragrant essences, savor the taste of food, and touch with pleasure the people and textures that surround our life. If we choose to, and if a partner is available to us, we explore our sensuality and sexuality with another. We are open, loving, and willing to share our self fully**. Body psychotherapy enhances our senses so that we are free to explore our sensuality and sexuality in our own way.**

Body Psychotherapy Reconnects Us to Our Soul

We meet with our body psychotherapist at the level of our soul. There is no judgment, shame, good or bad, weak or strong. There is only love, truth and pure connection. The forces that have kept us in a state of fear seem to miraculously lose their power and disappear. **Once we have experienced soul connection in a private body psychotherapy session, we can then go out into the world transformed, seeking that same soul connection with others.**

Body Psychotherapy Reminds Us To Play

We learn from a very early age the way the world is. Children play. Adults work. Children giggle. Adults are serious. Children feel emotions. Adults feel only a few acceptable emotions and repress the rest. Children are fully alive. Adults are careful and mature. In body psychotherapy, we discover we have choices about the way we want to live our life. We can choose to be serious, heavy-hearted, angry or depressed. Or we can lighten up and play and laugh at the absurdity of even the worst of our life circumstances and dilemmas. We begin to cherish the ever-present moment of now. **Body psychotherapy reminds us to lighten up, play, laugh and enjoy, from moment to moment, the simple pleasures of life.**

A Body Psychotherapy Session

For individuals, the first session involves an in-depth history. Couples, begin with a joint session, allowing both partners an equal opportunity to explain how they view their relationship issues and problems. At a later date, each partner returns privately for a history session. During the history sessions, I encourage clients to tell their personal stories in their own words. Scanning chronologically through the earlier years of their lives, we end by focusing on current relationship issues and what they hope to create in the future. Clients then have an opportunity to ask me how I work and what they might reasonably expect to experience in the therapy process.

Subsequent sessions are divided into a talking portion and a body therapy portion. Beginning with casual conversation about the past week and reactions to the previous session, any pressing issues or problems are brought out for discussion. When the salient issues have been addressed, at some point I will ask "Would you like to get on the table now?" Sometimes, clients are deeply involved in talking about something important and would prefer not to disrupt their train of thought. In such sessions, the bodywork may be delayed or there may be no body therapy at all.

When clients are ready to lie down on the body therapy table, they are asked to remove their shoes, glasses, and any bulky items in their pockets. Clients are never asked to remove any clothing! Once the client is lying on the body therapy table, I observe the tension points and breathing patterns. Slowly, carefully, and respectfully, I begin to approach touching.

Starting far from the center of my client's body, usually at the feet or head, I keep my palms a distance of about 12" above the body. Sitting quietly, allowing my own body to relax, I pay attention to the sensations between my hands. As I allow my hands to very slowly approach the surface of my client's body, I usually feel the heat and sensation of that person's energetic field. Depending on the physical and emotional state of the client's health, I may feel the sensation as far as 12" away or I may not feel it at all until my hands are actually touching the body.

Every client is unique. Every session is different. Sometimes I spend a long time at a person's feet, moving the legs, one at a time, rocking, shaking, stimulating meridian points and observing the movement from the leg into the hip joint and above. At other times, I spend a long time cradling a client's head in the palms of my hands or gently rocking it from side to side. I listen with my hands for places of restricted or easy movement. As I work, I continually look for changes in facial expressions and breathing.

Often, I check whether the person on the table feels comfortable and safe. **There is never, at any time, any contact with sexual organs or intimate body parts nor any touching for the purpose of sexual arousal.** Should the client express discomfort or a desire not to be touched at a specific time or in a particular place, I will always honor the client's request and immediately refrain from touching.

After the initial contact, I usually move closer to the center of the client's body. I may place one hand under the lower back and one hand gently resting on the abdominal area. This begins the energetic opening of the body through sustained holding with both of my hands. As I feel bodily tension diminish and the skin become tingly and warm, I may move my hands to another position, usually moving upwards to the rib cage, shoulders and neck, eventually cradling the head once again.

Sometimes I focus on opening the energy channels along specific acupressure meridians. At other times, or within the same session, I may do some gentle release techniques. These involve placing my hands under the client's hip, shoulder, or ankle, on one side of the body, to heighten awareness of the sensations in this body part. I will then slowly move my hands away as I feel the body part begin to let go of tension. Often, there is an obvious difference in the way this side of the body looks to my eye and feels to the client when compared to the opposite side of the body.

Differences in one side of the body compared to the other side, often leads to awareness of internal conflicts. At this point, we may begin some verbal dialogue. Depending upon the specific emotional and psychological issues that surface, movements (kicking, hitting, pounding fists) or emotional releases (crying, sighing, screaming) may spontaneously arise. To alleviate certain tension patterns, I sometimes guide the client's body to move into an unfamiliar and maybe uncomfortable position, perhaps a yoga posture, such as the fish or the cobra.

As the client's body releases chronically held tension, the logical, thinking mind may give way to a more intuitive, creative, non-linear way of thinking. Special chemicals in the brain and body cells, called neuropeptides, are released. New pathways are established in the complex body mind system. Images, memories, and powerful insights may emerge. New perspectives about life become integrated into ordinary thoughts and behaviors. **This is the miracle of body psychotherapy.**

Your Body's Messages

Sit quietly. Close your eyes. Take a few deep breaths and allow your body to relax. Pay attention to the changing thoughts in your mind. Notice whether any parts of your body feel uncomfortable, tense, painful, or seem to be calling for your attention. Pay attention. Continue to focus on the thoughts in your mind and the sensations in your body.

Think about the part or parts of your body that are in the foreground of your attention.

- *If these body parts could communicate, what sounds would they make?*

- *What colors would they be?*

- *What would be their quality or texture?*

- *Do the sensations you are currently feeling remind you of anything in nature or in your life?*

- *Is somebody or something in your life disturbing your emotional state?*

- *Are you causing your body to tighten or tense up in response?*

- *What messages about your life, your relationships, and your sexuality, are being offered to you by your bodily sensations?*

Body Psychotherapy Clears The Path For Love, Relationships And Intimacy

Our body reveals us to the world, to each other, and to our self. Through our energy and through touch, with or without words, we are known. As we discover that hiding is an illusion, we begin to relax our defenses. We discover that we are all longing to be accepted and loved. Scientists who study the universe, from the tiniest particles to the vastness of infinity, ultimately discover that love, attraction and repulsion rule the universe. **Through body psychotherapy, as we learn to love and accept our self and others, intimacy becomes our natural way of being.**

CONGRATULATIONS!

You have finished all the chapters in Book III. You have completed some powerful, life-transforming exercises. You have self-reflected about the ways that healing has occurred in your life. You have reviewed and contemplated how your thoughts, behaviors, attitudes and responses to the world and others' opinions may have blocked, interfered with, or enhanced your own healing process. You have discovered how powerful each of us really is and how important it is to tune in to your own inner knowing.

MORE TO COME!

LOVE ME … Please

Love Me … Please, the first book in this four part series, leads us on a path toward loving … truly loving, from the center of our being. Love is the ultimate aphrodisiac. Love is patient, kind, unyielding, enduring and steadfast. Love overcomes all obstacles. But what most of us have called love, our human concepts and human attempts at love, with its sense of limited supply, ownership, and "what's in it for me" attitude, is filled with illusion, self-consciousness, insecurity, doubt and emotional upheaval. True love, unconditional love, a higher state of love, is limitless, boundless, and the ultimate creative power of the universe.

This book is meant for lovers, people who love, people who want to love, people who have loved, and people who want to love again. You will not find simplistic answers and easy to follow formulas for creating love. You will have to look deep into your own consciousness – your thoughts, beliefs, attitudes, memories and dreams – to find the love, the fullest love, that you can bring into your life. And you will be reminded, over and over, to bring that love back to your own self so that you can fully share your loving self with others.

Touch Me ... Please

Touch Me ... Please introduces the healing potential of simple touch, from a gentle touch on the shoulder by an acquaintance, to the warm fuzzy feeling you get when your favorite pet cuddles us to you, or the wondrously tingly sensations of your intimate lover's touch.

This beautiful Ebook is sure to delight you with powerful real-life stories about the transformative power of touch, current research, abundant exercises for self-analysis and partner sharing as well as a full explanation of the wide variety of healing body therapies and healing somatic body psychotherapies.

Sexual and Spiritual Reawakening

We are all sexual. Sexuality teaches. Sexuality heals. Sometimes our sexuality hurts. When we allow our hearts to feel love and our bodies to feel pleasure, we are sexual. Being sexual is being alive. Feeling our sexual aliveness reawakens us to who we are. By allowing full sexual expression into our life, we cannot help but discover our spiritual nature.

We are also spiritual beings. Connecting to our spiritual nature and spiritual potential brings us an accepting appreciation of life. The path of discovering our spiritual connection can be difficult, painful and may reveal to us our deepest, darkest, most unloving personal attributes.

Our life path is a spiritual path, the process of rediscovering our connection to all that is. No matter which direction we choose to take, all paths will eventually lead us home. Every spiritual teaching reminds us of that simple truth. If we resist knowing this truth and pursue a self-centered and purely material way of life, we may encounter more struggle, more difficulties, and more tests than necessary. But even if we do pursue a spiritual path, there are still obstacles and difficulties to be overcome. The difference is that knowing our spiritual essence provides emotional strength and calmness in the face of any stormy life issues, problems and concerns. *Sexual and Spiritual Reawakening* is a simple guide to help you live a more fulfilling, life affirming and joyful existence.

Have any of the words or exercises in this book touched a sensitive place in your thoughts, emotions or beliefs?

Are you ready to Lose

- **Your fears?**
- **Your doubts?**

Are you ready to Create

- **Love and healing?**

It's NOT Too Late!

NOW IS THE TIME TO CREATE HEALING AND LOVE IN <u>YOUR</u> LIFE!

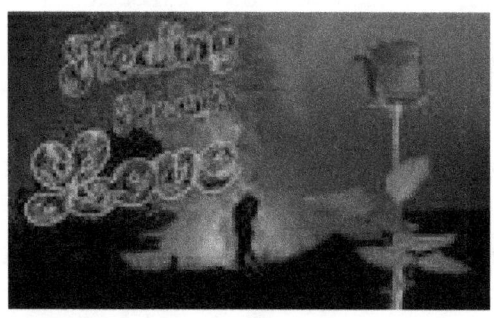

LoveNow.life/HealingThroughLoveSession

ALSO BY DR. ERICA GOODSTONE

KINDLE BOOKS

Beautiful Bare Feet: Fetish or Fantasy
Be Who You Are: The Greatest Gift of All
The Delicate Dance of Love
Your Body Believes You
It's a Sensational World
Touching Matters - The Profound Effects of Body Therapy
Let All Your Senses Speak – As You Heal
Touching Stories
Ordinary People, Ordinary Yet Extraordinary Sex
Sexual Reawakening: 10 Simple Steps
Sexual and Spiritual Reawakening – At Last!
The Science Of Being Well - Wallace D. Wattles author,
    Annotated and Illustrated by Dr. Erica Goodstone
The Science Of Getting Rich - Wallace D. Wattles author,
    Annotated and Illustrated by Dr. Erica Goodstone

Books and EBooks are available at
Amazon.com, Smashwords.com and Lulu.com

DIGITAL PROGRAMS

Love Touch Heal Video Series
Healing Through Love Audio Series
Love Lessons For Your Soul
Love Touch Heal Relationship Program

Copyright © 2009, Revised 2023   Heal Me … Please   DrEricaGoodstone.com

VIRTUAL SUMMITS

Men and Love Series
Women and Love Summit
Sexual Reawakening Summit
Love Me Touch Me Heal Me Summit
Healing Recovery Retreat
Miraculous Healing Master Class Summit
Science And Poetry of Love Summit
The Science of Being Well Docuseries

Programs, courses and summits available at
https://DrEricaGoodstone.com

AMAZON REVIEWS

If you have enjoyed reading this book, please consider leaving an Amazon review. The author will be most grateful because this enables her to reach more people who want to create more love in their lives.